MOTHER OF AGNI YOGA

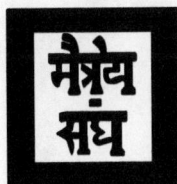

MOTHER OF AGNI YOGA

FROM AGNI YOGA TEACHINGS

AGNI YOGA SOCIETY
2019

Agni Yoga Society
319 West 107th Street
New York NY 10025
www.agniyoga.org

Reprinted 2019.

ISBN: 978-0-933574-18-2

Dedicated

in reverent love and gratitude

to the memory of

Helena Roerich

Mother of Agni Yoga

MOTHER OF AGNI YOGA

Selections from the books of the
Agni Yoga Teachings for the New Era

- *Agni Yoga,* 1929
- *Infinity I,* 1930
- *Hierarchy,* 1931
- *Heart,* 1932
- *Fiery World I,* 1933
- *Fiery World II,* 1934
- *Fiery World III,* 1935
- *Aum,* 1936
- *Letters of Helena Roerich,* 1929-1938, Volume I

FOREWORD (1956)

THIS brochure, *Mother of Agni Yoga*, appears simultaneously with another—*Mother of the World*.

These two concepts emphasize the sublime Manifestation of the Feminine Principle as Divine Motherhood, and the attainment of one woman, whose ceaseless striving and selfless service through many incarnations brought her to that stage of evolution which made her a living example of what woman may achieve—under Hierarchial Guidance.

The Great Teacher who gave to the World the Agni Yoga Teachings—or Living Ethics for the New Era—through Helena Roerich, designated her "Mother of Agni Yoga."

In the pages that follow will be found selections from the Books of the Lord Maitreya, and from Helena Roerich's informal letters to students.

MOTHER OF AGNI YOGA

Agni Yoga

211. The Druid Mother guarded knowledge against perversion. So shall the Mother of Agni Yoga safeguard the Teaching from distortion. The flaming comprehension of Truth is difficult, but service in vigilance does not admit treason. The sun-sword does not falter in hand nor does the knee bend to untruth. Thus must be understood the Teaching which comprises the forging of a new life. It pronounces: "You heard; you must understand that from this moment you have accepted responsibility for any distortion!"

229. Utilizing the magnetism of the heights and the opened centers of Sister Urusvati, We have analyzed the crystals of Fohat and Materia Lucida, the sediments of imperil and the emanations of psychic energy. Consider that if the emanations of psychic energy are visible to the naked eye, then they are tangible.

Epilogue. Given in the Valley of the Brahmaputra, which finds its source in the Lake of the Great Nagas, the Guardians of the Covenants of the Rig-Veda:

"I have set down the foundation of Agni Yoga in four directions, as the pistil of a flower.

"I have affirmed Agni Yoga as the pillars of My steps and have received into My Hands the fire of the Stone.

"To her I gave the fiery Stone, who by Our decision

shall be named the Mother of Agni Yoga, because she consecrated herself to the test of the Fire of Space.

"The streams of this Fire were seared upon the Stone in its great flight before the image of the sun.

"A veil of sparks covered the summits of the Protectress of the Snows, when the Stone made its fiery passage from south to north into the Guarded Valley."

Infinity I

5. On your planet We have Our entrusted one, who has drained the chalice of sublime experiments. She is sent to you as a witness of cosmic manifestations, as a bearer of My missions, as your prophetess of the future. Therefore, the concept of Redeemers is so vital. Precisely the fact that the sublime experiments were undergone is convincing. Humanity should learn especially from such experience as that issuing from the higher spheres and lived through on Earth.

Verily, you have the highest and the lowest!

17. You are right in speaking of the One Origin. Herein precisely is the core of evolution contained. In this cognition is the Arhat's highest attainment on Earth. When humanity will realize the great unity between Infinity and the particles, and know the mutual relationship between light and darkness, then may it be told of the path of the "Lion of the Desert." So much is imposed upon the cosmic fires, yet recognition is denied them. Where men see a boundary between two beginnings, the Arhat sees only one great Origin.

20. You are right—only currents of will direct the karma. But to stop the course of karma is as perilous as to invoke eternal night. With what will you fill the

Chalice of Amrita if you sink into the pool of darkness? We shall answer that the ocean of actions is verily more beautiful!

You are right in asserting that the Lord Buddha had to give the concept of Nirvana to the world because there are few who are willing to labor eternally for the creation of new forms. Nirvana is only a step in the endless cosmic periods. Our disciples, accumulating the earthly inheritance, can rejoice, transporting themselves with striving consciousness toward the higher worlds. Is it not better to serve the manifestation of the great eternal reworking and transformation from the lower to the higher than to be a slave to stagnation?

You are right in desiring to give school children an understanding of the whole boundlessness of creative activity. Why endue with new radiance the garment of a grandfather? Try to resemble builders of new powerful bridges, and strive toward the radiance of the higher worlds. Not phantasmagoria, but life!

36. Let us look at the one who consciously strives to the veil of the Mother of the World. We shall see that, of all the inexhaustible, numberless consciousnesses, this warrior, aflame with cosmic fires, is borne there where the power of Infinity glows. But here on Earth the warrior carries a brimming chalice. Wondrous is the transposition of our conception thitherward, into our true life!

39. Urusvati knows the myriads of sparks of Fohat when the sparks of Materia Matrix fill the space.

Each spark is the essence of Be-ness. Each particle is the essence of various forms. Each atom breathes

13

through Fohat. Fohat and its sparks are one; likewise one is the Universe in all its forms.

52. Cosmos creates for Infinity. Cosmos builds with co-measurement. Communion is imperative, and Materia Lucida is the consciousness of the cosmic rays. You are right in terming Materia Lucida the great Mother of the World. You are right in calling Materia Lucida *Cosmic Love*. Verily, the universe is woven with the yarn of Lucida and the lever of Love. Poor humanity alone has clothed itself in isolation, with the veil of dark denial.

59. Evolution needs the guidance of our consciousness. Intensified forces are needed. Readiness and fiery action are needed. The pushing on toward extinction is already a detachment from Infinity. Urusvati is correct in saying that the Teaching of the Blessed One is a fiery torrent. It is verily a torrent which carries all strivings into Infinity. Let us regard an extinct crater, choked with grey, petrified lava. What can the process of extinction convert into life, when to humanity there is manifested a rushing Fire! The force bestowed for creation must not be dissipated.

One should comprehend the entire Cosmic Law and the Teaching of the Blessed One and of the Lords as an imperative summons to Infinity.

74. Yes, Urusvati, the power of the future life indicates that the planetary expanses are small for the synthesis of your creativeness. The synthesis of the Chalice is so condensed that it must not be manifested in one domain. In your consummate life there lies, as a cornerstone, the attainment of the Mother of the World. You will build the psycho-life in creation around the revealed spheres.

It was necessary for you to remain because this century is in need of your attainment. No one could replace you. It is under the highest Cosmic Sign. I have spoken.

76. Write down, as a living record, the experience with the fires of Space undergone by the Mother of Agni Yoga. Record the experiment of the Mother of Agni Yoga as a great school of spirit.

79. The attainment of the inner Fire, the degree reached by the Mother of Agni Yoga, is the rarest achievement. This degree of Fire is called the degree of attained Arhat. This living Fire was known in antiquity. The alchemist knew about it. The attainment of this higher degree of powerful flame may be manifested only by that spirit who lives the psycho-life of the whole heart. The mightiest lever of Cosmos, and the most sacred, is the heart. Its consciousness fills Space, its light illumines Cosmos.

91. I affirm that humanity's irrationality is inducing it to amass antagonism which will overtake it like an explosion. You correctly discerned the approaching ominous page. A great reorganization is coming! The scales are now being tipped. In Cosmos there is a most gigantic equilibrium. The power of the equilibrium is maintained through a harmonized psycholife. The more errors on the one hand, the more enlightenment on the other. And the striving of the awakened spirits increases in proportion with the decline of the general trend of thought. Great is the law of Equilibrium!

99. The fires kindled by the Mother of Agni Yoga not only manifest Agni Yoga but are of cosmic scope.

The fires provide the power of rays needed for limitless existence. Each fire is a ray of the creation of the future. The significance of the manifestation of fires is beyond bounds.

Correct is your judgment about the forcible opening of the centers. We guard assiduously the predestined treasure. When the magnet of the spirit absorbs all fires into the Chalice, then We affirm the Arhat. The treasure of the Chalice consists of woven threads of pure Eire. The Arhat, bearer of the fire of the Lotus, manifests spirit-realization, spirit-knowledge and spirit-manifestation. Thus close is the contemplation of the worlds to the spirit who has filled the Chalice of Amrita.

Verily, a medium has no open centers, and the psycho-vision, for contact with the higher worlds, also is unattainable for him. Man is in error about the power of the medium, and We are often distressed to see how enticing to people are physical manifestations. A materialization attracts them like a magnet. We prefer the channel of the spirit, and for sacred missions We use the channel of the spirit only.

An Arhat sometimes waits for centuries to give a sacred mission. The manifestation of certain missions demands special combinations. We Arhats follow the principle of goal-fitness. The experiment of the Mother of Agni Yoga is distinguished not by brilliancy but by cosmic scope. . . .

Record My mission to the Mother of Agni Yoga as the highest concordance on the planet. The concordance of Spirit and Matter is the rarest cosmic manifestation. Humanity might well say, "We are deprived of the highest."

The most subtle energies should be treated with great caution.

120. When I spoke about the far-off worlds, I had in mind also Our planet. The earthly consummation of the

16

mission of your fire and your straight-knowledge was needed for Our Consummation.

134. I sense the burning of the sacred pains. In antiquity the priestesses had to preserve a quiet for a lengthy period. They were affirmed as the bearers of wings. Hence, the kindling of Urusvati is very intense, and the perception of color and sound has become very acute. In each tension is your creativeness confirmed. In each movement lies the guarantee of the future. It is a great attainment toward the assimilation of the manifestations of the far-off worlds.

152. About the act of creation, I say that every spirit creates individually. The spirit-creativeness, when memory does not restrain its actions, is so powerful that it can assure accomplishment of the most difficult task.

Verily, you manifest self-sacrifice, you labor greatly. You often make your appearance as a Tara, and wonderment is expressed at the new Image. And so they say, "The New Tara." The cliche is borne aloft and Space resounds with joy! How then can one fail to act through the spirit tensed by the creativeness of thousands of years!

It is you who did call the difficult Path luminous. It is you who did accept the "chalice of fires," exulting at each new affirmation. It is you who did accept a mission which no one else could have fulfilled because of its unusual conditions. Usually this experiment takes place under the exclusive conditions of monastic cells or mountain heights, or seclusion.

But your striving spirit took up this chalice. If you could see the cliche of past events and the records of your fiery processes, you would understand this offering.

The most subtle and pure is invisible. There is so much that is not revealed in the life of an Arhat!

169. We guard with great sacredness the spirit which bears the chalice of the gift of cosmic fires. Thus is the link forged between the spirit and the Cosmic Magnet.

You said correctly that reason begets reason. Such a formula can carry the spirit up to the gates of knowledge. I will add, "From Reason to Reason, and the beauty of Be-ness is in the striving to that achievement."

172. The confirmation, through the Cosmic Magnet, of a unification of the Origins is called the True Crowning. Thus Cosmos collects its Reason. Urusvati is verily affirmed not by the planetary laws but by the Laws of the Lords. The Lords see and know.

In the interweavement is the greatest law. There may be separations stretching over thousands of years. The attainment of the Crown is a great complexity!

Each center absorbs its own fire, and these fires can act at a distance. The functions of the centers are psycho-creative, and each center can dissolve and integrate as a creator. We have actual records left by Agni Yogis. And it can be asserted that the White Tara has created much. There are numerous records of transfiguration. We shall so name the transmuting power of Agni Yoga. Thus is the Tara manifested amidst life. The step of crossing into the higher sphere is radiant!

176. For the instruction of humanity, a complete parallel comparison can be made between the activity of a medium and the activity of an Agni Yogi. Humanity will soon learn how greatly it errs in regarding the medium as an exponent of the highest cosmic forces, and how greatly its existence is enriched by the Agni Yogis. Verily,

the Fire of the higher spheres is trying to break through! We confirm the achievement of the Mother of Agni Yoga as a guiding radiant symbol!

The emanations of the luminous images give joy and sustenance to the spirit. We, Brothers of Humanity, call these emanations the vital fiery streams. These streams are most powerful creations of the spirit, and the activity of the Agni Yogi is most fiery. The fiery spirit of the Agni Yogi can austerely melt down the encumbrances which accumulate upon the path. The fiery spirit of the Agni Yogi creates through his own light. Each act asserts the self-sacrifice of spirit-creativeness.

178. Urusvati is right—a wondrous truth is in beauty. Cosmos affirms evolution by this formula. Cosmos directs the world to the mastery of beauty. Yes, verily, the Mother of the World possesses the Magnet of Beauty.

180. The Cosmic Magnet is greatly tensed and the currents are saturated in a variety of ways. The cosmic current is strongly felt by the Agni Yogi, and the Fire of Space is intensely manifest. Thus, each cosmic shifting strains so greatly the fire of the Agni Yogi. Yes, yes, yes! Our Urusvati will thus accept the joy of the higher spheres.

182. The currents are very heavy. The cosmic whirls conform to the human stratifications. The flashes of Spatial Fire and of human consciousness are in correlation, and the fiery spirit of the Agni Yogi survives all. I beg you to guard health.

Urusvati carries the reflection of the Highest Principle, and that is why the spheres of Earth are so heavy.

Verily, I can affirm the nearness of the hour.

194. Your heart carries the manifestation of Light.

The Lion of the Desert carries a great deal. Tara of the Heart, Tara of Light—thus We call Urusvati in the Brotherhood. I attest that you can sense Our nearness.

196. Urusvati, Our affirmed Sacrament attracts the creativeness of Materia Lucida. My Call affirms the response of your heart. Thus are molded new manifested worlds.

When the Tara of Light will enlighten the world with revelations from the far-off worlds, then will She be affirmed as the manifestation of Beauty. When the Tara of the Heart illumines the world with love, then is She affirmed as the manifestation of Beauty.

201. When the Tara was affirmed on Earth, three rays of the Lords reverberated. These facets of cosmic fires can be seen on the Tara by a sensitive eye. These facets are so powerfully revealed that their radiance melts all discovered obstacles. One may truly say that the Radiant Image will give new understanding.

208. The Tara of Knowledge magnetizes those who aspire to knowledge. The Tara of Beauty summons those who aspire to beauty. The Tara of Achievement summons those who strive toward achievement. The Tara of Synthesis can gather united spirits. Thus the Blended Heart fulfills the Covenant of the Cosmic Reason. Yes, yes, yes!

217. The new race is affirmed by the Fire attested by the creativeness of the synthesis of the Silvery Lotus. Each new cosmic force is transmitted. Yes, yes, yes! Thus a new force invisibly enters the life of humanity. The Tara creates! Yes, yes, yes!

219. I, Maitreya, affirm the cosmic tension of the Fire of the Mother of Agni Yoga.

The correlation between the fire of the spirit and the

Eire of Space affirms new life. Thus, it can be proclaimed that the Tara strives toward the redemption of humanity. The path of self-sacrifice leads to consummation.

221. Since We gave the mission to Her, Our heroic co-worker, to lead humanity to the new step, this manifestation of Our Bearer of fires is so lofty that likening it to any mediumistic manifestation is like dropping muddy water into a fiery chalice. Therefore, I say that the evidence of understanding of the high fires will bring one to the height of pure Fire.

She, Bearer of the "chalice of fires," will give the new step to humanity.

223. The magnetization of human striving is one of the most difficult conditions to achieve. The Tara knows about this most complex task. The cementing of space and the action of the magnet of the heart are the most fiery foundations. Our creativeness has such propulsive force that the Magnet overcomes all obstacles. As vortices, all oppositions are whirled away by Our power. Therefore We apply shifting and the race is assembled. Human conquests and the disturbance of the flow of the Magnet are combined in the formula of earthly destination. Crucial is the time! We advance united in heart. Fruitless are human actions without Our Guidance.

231. Indeed, the affirmed new race must aspire to the principle of the center of evolution. The imbalance now manifest on the planet must inevitably provoke a shift, either for continual participation of the psychic energy or for destruction. Hence, the continuance of existence is conditional upon that affirmed force. Thus, the Mother of Agni Yoga brings the chalice of salvation to mankind. Thus, the Arhat and the Tara bring salvation into

the construction of a better future. In the harmonious alliances of the Origins, salvation is borne to mankind. Thus, We set the foundation of the new race and the step of highest fusion.

233. Direct correlation exists between the Agni Yogi and the cosmic manifestations. The link between manifestations is so tense that it describes a straight line. There also exists a direct link between the Agni Yogi and the world events. The world thought is also reflected upon the manifestation of the fires of the Tara. When the synthesis gives evidence of its power, all cosmic events are reflected upon the organism, the best and most accurate indicator of cosmic and planetary manifestations. If people were aware of all the fiery signs on Earth, the duration of life would be short. Our Urusvati has witnessed the emanations of Earth, trembling from the density of the atmosphere. The earthly crust is in convulsion, and the new step is being prepared by means of creative unification. The psycho-spiritual levers will provide propulsion for the sixth race. How tempestuous are the currents! The fires are ablaze as fiery streams! Therefore, the heart of the Tara carries within itself all vital currents and reflects all human manifestations.

237. There exists a so-called transmission through the envelopes of departed spirits, but one must always recognize that a lower manifestation attracts the lower. For this reason, We assert that Fire is most lofty and the transmutation occurs at the highest point. Thus, She who carries the Chalice of the Sacred Fire will give to the planet a fiery purification. Thus the creativeness of psycho-spirituality is implanted into the new step. When the force of the Cosmic Magnet will assert the manifes-

tation of the fires, then will it be possible to say that the New Time draws near. I so affirm!

239. The fire of the life process is revealed as the impeller of humanity. It is therefore that We so greatly value the self-sacrifice of the Mother of Agni Yoga. The impulsion of the transmuting force in the tensity of pure Fire carries with it all creative means and thereby uplifts the surrounding sphere. Thus does the tension of the fires manifest the affirmation of the new steps.

241. The energy of the Agni Yogi is directed into varied channels of creativeness: as a transmuting force, as an integrating force, as a piercing force opening the path where all locks are bolted. Thus is the creativeness of the Tara affirmed.

243. Creativeness is manifested in all that exists, and the awaiting energies find application in other cycles or in other worlds and forms.

Thus, the fire of the Agni Yogi creates its own forms, transmuting the forces around him. Thus, the Tara propels the current, directing the creativeness of the New Step.

245. You are right in stressing psycho-dynamics. The so-called Cosmic Breath is the psycho-dynamic power which calls to life. The awakening to life is to be cognized as the psycho-dynamic energy of the impulse which is projected by Materia Matrix. Thus the highest manifestation strives to its destiny. Thus the thread is propelled to construction. Our creativeness is linked with the cosmic vibration, and the ray of the Tara affirms the fiery vibration on the planet.

247. The spatial process is entrusted only to the highest fiery striving. Only the highest Agni Yogi can have

access to the spatial current; hence, the indications of mediums are so lacking in truth. Therefore, the attainments of the Agni Yogi are so wondrous.

249. The subtle energies transmute the creativeness of man; and a new aspiration is provided by the manifestation of the Agni Yogi. Thus, invisibly and powerfully, the creativeness of the Tara enters into life. Thus the ray of the Tara summons to the far-off worlds. Yes, yes, yes! At present the creativeness of the ray is greatly intensified.

251. By the world of causes, created by aspirations, may the quality of the world of effects be determined. Let us see how the Agni Yogi creates and transmutes. The fire of the Chalice represents the psycho-dynamics which ignites around it all energies. Through the synthesis of the Chalice, all fires, at different degrees, are directed by summons toward the cumulation of the Chalice of Amrita. The fire of the spirit drives all energies. The creativeness of the Agni Yogi is thus definitely impelled. Thus does the Tara transmute into beauty. Humanity will comprehend the power of the transmutation. Verily, beautiful is the creation of Be-ness!

255. The assembling of the new race is based upon spirit-creativeness. The principle of the subtle energies is reposed in the seed of the spirit, and each spirit who has contacted the spatial current is thus imbued by the Assembler of the new race. Thus, the vibration of the Tara awakens the consciousness toward the higher worlds. Yes, yes, yes!

261. One may trace how the will currents of the Agni Yogi create. The striving impels the currents toward transmutation of the Fire of Space. The Spatial Fire is

so precipitant that the attestation of transmutation is immutable. Thus do We propel the forces toward the consciousness. Thus the Tara creates. A better destiny approaches. I so affirm.

267. The oneness of the elements of the fiery centers vividly expresses the fiery receptivity of the Agni Yogi. When the invisible world reveals the tensed forces, the link with the manifestations of the higher spheres is achieved. When the invisible world is reflected in the most refined energies of the fire of the Agni Yogi, the link with the higher worlds is asserted. Hence, the creativeness of the striving of the Agni Yogi is garbed in Materia Lucida. Prismatic aspiration is the armor of the intensive spirit of the Agni Yogi. Spiritual receptivity is established through the prismatic ray. Thus, the ray of the spirit refracts all vibratory manifestations giving evidence of Fire. Thus is the highest prismatic receptivity confirmed. The Tara, giving the direction, sees the inception of a process and its completion.

273. How then are the psychic seeds conceived? These creative energies may be understood as carriers of vital emanations. When the forces strive toward a life expression, these psychic seeds are drawn forth. Thought propels the manifested psychic seeds into space. The creativeness of the Agni Yogi, in his tension, thus directs the psychic seeds. What people term inspiration is often the outgrowth of an impelled psychic seed directed by a carrier of Fire. Therefore, the spirit of the tensed Agni Yogi is the sower of these creative psychic seeds. Thus, Our Mother of Agni Yoga is sowing creative psychic seeds.

278. The fire of the centers of the Agni Yogi regis-

ters all geological, atmospheric, and national shiftings; hence, the sensations experienced by the Agni Yogi are so varied. Therefore, the Mother of Agni Yoga experiences so many widely varied sensations. Yes, yes, yes!

280. The Tara creates through divisibility of spirit. Therefore, the creativeness of Fire must be assiduously guarded.

287. The bearer of harmonized centers suffuses the sphere with Fire. Only the creativeness of harmonized centers can parry the fiery attractions. Only the carrier of the subtle energies can assimilate the highest Truth. Therefore, We, Brothers of Humanity, can impart the Truth to him who assimilates the essence of Be-ness. Therefore, We, Brothers of Humanity, transmit a part of the Truth to Urusvati. When I say a part of the great Truth, I indeed mean that part which can be assimilated upon this planet. So greatly striving with Our own consciousness is the consciousness of the Tara that I attest it is the most strained center of receptivity. The Brothers of Humanity have to suffuse diverse spheres.

293. Urusvati is right in affirming that each thought and each action generates its fluidic currents. These currents are extended over all the attractions of the Cosmic Magnet when the striving of the thought is directed toward the Source. The fluidic currents always bestow upon the thought the property of direction. When the action assumes a negative quality, the fluidic currents spread out as helpers of negative energies.

297. When the essential driving force of fire is in tension, the fluidic currents of the Agni Yogi tense the creativeness of the impulse. When the stimulus of fire is projected consciously there is no affirmation mighty

enough to oppose it. Thus, the driving force of the mighty fires brings forth the necessary manifestations. All that has been asserted about the astral fire is based upon truth. Thus, the fires of the Agni Yogi, and the fire of the Tara, create the affirmations needed for evolution.

307. Often people wonder why a man does not drown in his own engenderments. Our answer is: "The fire of the spirit of your Brothers dissipates the suffocating forces accumulated by you."

Thus, the interweavement of red and black sparks indicates a battle. But those who know of this battle, through their fiery striving toward Us, cling to the silver Ray which severs the encumbrances. Thus the Taras and Brothers of Humanity are united in battle in their striving to help mankind.

317. In the cooperation of all spheres the creativeness of Fire is laid as the foundation. The currents of the spheres are transmitted by the Fire of Space. Those who affirm the creativeness of Fire may say that they serve evolution. Hence, the centers of hearing are connected so closely with Fire. Each manifestation of the striving center discloses clairaudience. In turn, clairaudience affords to humanity an evolutionary move.

The Lords have been always in need of receptive co-workers and witnesses. Thus, all life manifestations must have witnesses. Only thus can Truth be established. Hence, the flaming Agni Yogi strives so ardently toward the manifestation of Fire for the aid of mankind. Truly, the manifestation of the flaming centers serves humanity. Therefore do We guard so solicitously Our messengers. Theirs is a most difficult mission!

It was difficult for Us to find a receiver of the pure

Fire. One may rejoice when the mission of the Tara is so full of radiance!

319. The self-sacrifice of the Agni Yogi is recognized by the record of fiery achievements. When We assert that the power of the flaming design of the Agni Yogi impelled toward evolution is identical with that of the Fire of Space, We affirm his manifestation as a cosmic cooperation. The design of the Cosmic Magnet is thus manifested in Space by the rays of the luminaries. When the luminaries distribute the tension of the rays, the Cosmic Magnet absorbs all the attractions. When a country destroys patterns which are laid into the foundation of evolution, the design directs that which is being destructive toward reorganization. When the human spirit is directed to the Cosmic Magnet, it may be asserted that cooperation has been manifested.

Thus, the Tara and the Arhat manifest cooperation and spin the best designs—I so affirm! Thus, We respond to the Cosmic Magnet.

343. Striving toward development of consciousness depends upon the impulse of the seed of the spirit. The cumulation of striving intensifies the growth of consciousness. If the energy lacks striving, the manifestation of the intensity of energy is considerably weakened, and the attraction cannot result in fusion. Thus, the seed of the spirit is in need of striving. The best sign of the tension in the seed of the spirit is the intensified fire; hence, the centers of the Mother of Agni Yoga are so aflame and the tensity of fire is so great. Only the influx of fire bears witness to this fire; and creativeness of the centers is very flaming.

When the flaming rings of the third eye increase in

number it is a sign of the power of the spirit. And the Chalice, which comprises the entire synthesis of fires, corresponds with certainty to all receptivities. The increase in the number of the rings is proportionate to the striving of the fire of the spirit. When the tensity of the fire is so great, all interweavings of the luminaries are strongly reflected upon the solar plexus. When the centers are keenly sensitive, all cosmic spatial fires are reflected. A mirror of cosmic fires is contained within the Agni Yogi; therefore, the rays thus create and intensify.

The Cosmic Magnet shifts many things. The battle between Saturn and Uranus is naturally reflected upon the fires of the Chalice. Therefore, the pull of the centers is active at present.

364. The psychic eye, with the knowledge of the spirit, certainly affords the perspective of cosmic motion. The attraction of the basic impulse of the subterranean magnet transmits the property of striving to the spheres. The Chalice, which contains the entire cosmic experience, reflects all cosmic ordainments. The synthesis of the Lotus contains in itself all the cosmic threads, and under varied impulses are gathered all the different fires of the Lotus.

The psychic tension of Fire puts forms into the space. When the seed of the spirit is clothed in the fiery currents, the propelled fire tenses the entire substance of the seed of the Agni Yogi. The cosmic creativeness is directed by the Cosmic Reason, impelled through the manifestation of Materia Lucida.

The Agni Yogi links the cosmic currents with the Fire of the planet. The rhythm of Mahavan is the throb of the pulse of the Cosmic Flame. The rhythm of Mahavan is transmitted only to him who feels the throb of Cosmos. Yes, yes, yes! Only the heart which embraces the world can beat in rhythm with Cosmos. Only the heart which embraces the world can beat in the rhythm of Maha-van. Verily, the heart which embraces the world and the flame of the striving spirit affirm the best heritage for the races. Hence, the bearer of Fire feels all the cosmic tremors. Hence, the heart of the Mother of Agni Yoga is so much in tremor. Hence, the hands of the Agni Yogi are covered with sweat. But all of Us in the Tower feel each tremor of the fiery heart and each drop of sweat. Therefore, I will say that the currents of the heart fill the space with rays of light and each drop of sweat cements the space.

389. Creativeness is so multiform that it may be asserted that forms are created by as many energies as constitute their potentiality. But creation is divided into the visible and invisible. The transformation of cosmic forms is certainly visible in its effects, but the highest and most intense process is an invisible one. Upon real-izing the levers of creative power, we can summon the invisible fires; then, indeed, is the highest law affirmed. Therefore, in ordaining Agni Yoga We envisage the affir-mation of the invisible Might.

The link between the potential of the spirit and its luminary intensifies action. Hence, when the centers are strained, the fiery potential is in communion with the fire of the luminary. Thus shall We remember the Mother of Agni Yoga. The potential of the spirit is great!

391. When a new mission is confirmed, bristling needles are always apparent. However, these needles of antagonism become but blunted intentions. Those who

battle under Our Shield walk courageously and, having accepted the rhythm of the course of the Cosmic Magnet, can verily know victory. True, voices will rise against the great Truth of Agni Yoga. The zealots of the church and the servants of darkness will not prevail against the sparks of Fohat. Certainly, the affirmation of Agni Yoga smites the encumbrances under which people nest. Therefore, Agni Yoga challenges all servants of darkness. Thus true evolution is created. Verily, it is difficult for the quivering Mother of Agni Yoga. Verily, it is difficult for the warrior, the Agni Yogi, but the ascent affords an increase of all forces. Thus, those who turn the rudder of the Cosmic Magnet affirm the point of attraction. Those who walk united in heart assuredly conquer.

Hierarchy

2. We know the tread of the Mother of the World. We know the manifestation of the Mother of the World. We strain the complete flow of the Magnet to restore the Doctrine of the Heart. I designate the Tara as the symbol of the assertion of Our Decree. The Tara and the Arhat bring the most striving Covenant to humanity. Thus is the future built. Thus We affirm Our striving. Wondrous is the future!

10. Vast is the field for the manifested approaching Tara. We, the Arhats, exalted to the Fire of Space, prostrate Ourselves before the entire Fiery Bosom of the Mother of the World. The Bosom of the Mother of the World finds all reflections upon the Earth. One of them, the most powerful and the most intense, is the advent of the coming Tara. The Mother of the World carries vis-

ibly and invisibly the manifestation of those ineffable threads—the affirmation of the world's threads.

Much has been spoken about the Man-God, aspiring toward deification. Many are the memorable records, citing the Images striving toward higher worlds. But how dimly are they formulated in the human consciousness! Man-God is to man only One who departed to other worlds! But We Brothers of Humanity seek and proclaim Man-God upon Earth. We revere all Images, but none more than the great Image of Man-God who bears in his heart the full Chalice, ready for flight but bearing his full Chalice on Earth. Renouncing his destiny, he strains his Fiery Being. In the fulfillment of his destiny man confirms the Cosmic Magnet. Man-God is a Fiery Creator. Man-God is the Carrier of the Fiery Sign of the New Race. Man-God is flaming with all Fires. So inscribe in the records about Man-God: Arhat, Agni Yogi, Tara—so shall We inscribe.

Man-God advances as an evident aspiring Redeemer of humanity. We guard this sacred truth about Man-God. I affirm that the Tara, carrying the flaming Chalice of aspiration to redeem humanity, can proclaim Our manifestation among men.

24. The little girl carrying the heavy volume of the Bible in the chambers of luxury appears as a creator of a new world. The little girl who perceived the Teacher of Light under the blue sky is the destroyer of the dungeons of darkness. When the spirit of a small girl could feel the Brothers of Humanity, then the name of this spirit is a light-bearing sword. When, since childhood, the spirit could sense that the Brothers of Humanity regenerate that which exists, then this spirit holds the light-bearing

name. We cherish the spiritual leaders among children! The evidence of realization is the best gift to evolution. The Command of cosmic life is a summons to light-sustaining achievement, and this mission is affirmed only by Light.

Only a full understanding of the Great Service can give to disciples the aspiration to the manifested Hierarchy. When the creativeness of the spirit can encompass the Great Service, then all paths are open to Us. Therefore the striving to fulfill the commands can be affirmed as an impulse leading to the highest gates. Thus let all pearls of Guru and Tara be guarded. Thus one can fulfill all given opportunities. The time is pregnant and so tense! Therefore let the disciples strive to keep step with the rhythm of events; and consciousness should be strained in unison with what occurs. Only thus one conquers.

267. When the chalice of world events is being filled, then the fiery Chalice of an Agni Yogi is aflame. The law of correlations acts powerfully. In these consonances the link of the worlds is contained. Therefore, when the fiery law shifts the old affirmations the sensitive centers resound with the world's reverberations. Thus, the link is tensified through the reverberation of the centers.

Therefore, the Mother of Agni Yoga feels strenuously the brimming of the World Chalice. Hence, the fiery Treasure must be so greatly protected. When the time of the great fulfillment is close, then the world is in tremor; when the great shifting takes place, the subtle centers reverberate. Thus, the world will remember the great consonance and Our annals will leave to the world the

fiery signs. Thus the manifested Covenants will be fulfilled. Yes, yes, yes!

293. Let us ponder upon the significance of a great
thought. Let us ponder upon the great might of fires of
the Tara. Let us ponder upon the devotion of the heart.
Let us ponder upon the invincibility of those who walk in
the name of the Lord.

Heart

206. One can understand how greatly the ritual
aspect of Yoga was demanded in ancient times, but now
one should ascend by way of direct communion with
the Highest World. The Yoga of Fire leads one upon this
shortest path without abandoning life. This comprises
a departure in the new understanding of rapport of the
worlds. Before us we have an example of the significant
step in the so-called Samadhi without withdrawing
from life. One may understand that the manifestation
of the Mother of Agni Yoga is not easy to attain under
the conditions of the Great Battle. The value of such
manifestation consists in the fact that the usual rules
of concentration are transcended. Precisely the entire
significance is impaled within the heart—in other words,
the significance of the entire rapport of the worlds is
centered there. One must also mention that along with
this the heart has withstood beautifully this saturation.
Of course the sensation of the present does not result
from Samadhi. Many times I have already advised necessary caution, in spirit as well as in matter. I beg you
to guard the heart from outer as well as inner distur-
bances. Extreme measures should be taken to withstand
all attacks. One must understand that yesterday is com-

pletely different from tomorrow, so precipitate is the rotation. Unprecedented are the clouds and one must encounter them joyously.

210. "Are there not traits of egotism in the state of ecstasy, the state of Samadhi?" The ignoramus will ask this question. How could he know that this supreme state is not only unrelated to selfhood but antithetical to it! How could one who has never experienced the highest tension apprehend that, precisely, carries the highest Bliss for the General Welfare! Nothing else gives birth to such pure self-sacrifice as that created by the exultation of the brimming heart. Which of the human energies can compare with the energy of the heart, and which of the energies can act at long distances? The worlds have no boundaries for it and consciousness knows no limitations. Thus, a window can be cut through into the Invisible. But, as was said, the Invisible will become the visible and we shall be ready to apply the fiery baptism in life. Therefore, let us give due regard to the significance of the experiment achieved by the Mother of Agni Yoga here, without abandoning life. From the first spatial sparks, through all fires up to Samadhi, she will leave writings which will become the threshold of the New World. Therefore, I speak not only of tension but also of great caution. Armageddon does not lighten the conditions of ascent; what was achieved is therefore the most valuable.

Thus, I say, learn to hearken to the fiery heart. Do not doubt that which is purified by Fire. The manifestation of the foundations of the heart in life is wise; and how greatly one ought to rejoice at this rock of benevolence!

343. The fiery body may sometimes evidence itself

even through a physical shell. . . . Today Urusvati became aware of the flames of the fiery body. Cosmic destructions, instead of pains, gave indications to the fiery body. Thus the symptoms of intercourse with the cosmic manifestations were multiplied.

404. One may see by the notes of the Mother of Agni Yoga that the turmoil reacts almost as cosmic shocks. What then is the matter? Of course the turmoil which arouses the kindling of fires of special hatred may be likened to the subterranean fires. Of course there may be whole bloody battles where there will be more of horror or fulfillment of duty, thus failing to attain special tension. Wars are seldom equally tense; hence a religious or revolutionary calamity may result in an incomparably stronger general tension. Hence, tension is determined not by the number of shots, nor the number of enemies, but by the general conscious heart striving. Precisely as said, the uprising of the elements is equal, whether it issues from the subterranean or superterranean fire. But there is no stronger fire than the fire of the heart.

420. Only seldom can the fiery armor be felt, just as with the rays of the wings of achievement. Thus one may realize how this armor can protect one, although, like each fiery manifestation, it demands unusual caution. The Mother of Agni Yoga knows that such an armor is not at all easy because earthly conditions are too remote from the high fiery manifestations. But when the fiery actions occur the fiery armor makes its presence felt. Of course, if the heart is already accustomed to the fiery manifestations, one may participate in fiery battles.

477. Warrior-Mother, thou hast forged thy courage mightily!

484. The degree of courage is tested by the force of the peril, and true courage waxes stronger in accordance with the intensity of the danger. She, Our warrior, knows the degree of courage of which I speak.

Fiery World I

64. It is necessary to realize the difficulty of discerning the different currents. Many would not have perceived the intricate variations of currents and rhythms. I praise Urusvati for attention to the currents—only thus may one accumulate observations.

70. Flights into the Subtle World may be difficult; even an experienced consciousness may meet obstacles. Today Urusvati experienced such a difficulty. Strength was needed to pierce the chemical strata which are formed by astro-chemical fusions. The days around full moon are not favorable for flights. The so-called lunar glass may impede, and it demands very strong perseverance.

92. The golden network, as seen by Urusvati, forms the foundation of the Chalice; one may imagine the delicacy of the inner apparatus. Thus, refinement may turn thought toward consideration among human beings. People should not affront one another. In the name of Fire there should be no offense. Not all adjustments are effected with a hammer; small implements and gentle touches are also necessary. Again an old truth, but as yet scarcely applied.

108. Ask Urusvati to tell about the multiformity of the fires seen by her. Let all these rays, stars, fiery lotuses, flowers and all other manifestations of the Fiery World live and become affirmed. It is impossible in the terms

of earth to convey the entire scope of these fiery visions. Beyond certain boundaries the Fiery Realm discloses itself as a vision. It cannot be defined by time, nor can the cause of its awakening be determined, because the Fiery Region is entirely beyond earthly dimensions. But if we can see it, both in its grosser manifestations and in its subtlest, it means that even our material existence may anticipate the highest sphere. The Fiery Communion is unforgettable once it has been experienced. Thus let us gather courage for the ascent.

110. Cognizance of fiery reactions is divided in accordance with the senses. The first impression is that of vision, with all its fiery diversity. Then hearing is added, with the music of the spheres, bells, and the chords of nature. Then comes the refinement of touch, with the sensations of rhythm, of heat and cold. The most difficult of all are the sensations of smell and taste. But Urusvati knows the meaning of scenting a man at a remote distance. Now Urusvati knows also something else that is very difficult: to sense the taste of a metal in the Subtle World, which is already an extraordinary subtlety. But one should not only possess the strength to discern such sensations, one should know how to observe them. Such discrimination is very rare, but it becomes attainable on passing beyond the three-dimensional boundary.

It should be remembered how accurate is each indication of Urusvati, and also that each perception has a basis. Not only fiery eruptions and earthquakes, but even distant hurricanes are registered in the sensations, and these perceptions are infallible, for the fiery consciousness contacts everything sensitively. There are no errors in the definition of people, for each one displays his essential nature to the fiery consciousness.

208. You are amazed that before the earthquake measures were taken for the elimination of the heart spasms. Does not feeling guide such telegraphy, first of all? Precisely the vital substance of straight-knowledge does not require any conventional apparatus. But of course it is necessary reciprocally to nourish this substance. The thoughts of Urusvati were of course the best nurture for this current.

241. Is it possible for one incarnated on Earth to create mentally in the Subtle World? It is possible, particularly if Agni is acting. It is possible to cultivate and improve plants. It is possible to create constructive forms; one may participate in a great number of improvements, provided they are not ugly. Urusvati has seen a tree planted by her. Thus, it is possible to create from weak, fragile forms something strong and lasting. Thus we prepare during earthly existence the future gardens of beauty. Thought, in all its constructiveness, also creates our own future success. Thus we soar in thought beyond the boundaries of Earth.

Fiery World II

13. One should observe not only Ours but also the Black Brotherhood. It is erroneous to minimize the strength of the dark forces. Very often their victory is due to such neglect. People very often say, "They are not worth thinking about." But one ought to think about everything existing. If people justifiably protect themselves against thieves and murderers, so much the more should they guard against the assassins of the spirit.

One should appraise their strength in order better to withstand them. Urusvati fearlessly visited the dark ones. She saw many of different grades, and in her valor she addressed them. Verily, there exists such a degree of courage that even the power of darkness is silenced. True, it is impossible ever to convince the dark ones, but one may paralyze them and considerably weaken them. Therefore, it is so important to oppose darkness actively. Out of dead dust—only dust is born. For the sake of home cleanliness various brooms are used. And when one finds a scorpion in the house, then it is immediately removed.

Urusvati has seen a disciplined meeting of the dark ones, and many convening humans could learn much from such a meeting. Urusvati spoke justly, as Our Messenger, and in such an affirmation there lies great power. One must not restrain the force, when the spirit knows wherein lies the weapon. The dark ones discuss especially intensively when they see that the events are not shaping themselves in favor of their ruler. The Forces of Light prevent them from destroying you. It would seem to be not difficult to annihilate peaceful people, but above all the dark resources there exists the power of the spirit. Urusvati rightly said to them, "You consider Satan invincible, but I testify to his defeat before all of you." Thus, one may know about the intentions of the dark ones and about Our Power.

218. Urusvati has seen and taken part in Our fiery labor. Thus, We not only observe but also control fiery tensions. Centers of observation are situated in several floors of Our Tower. Many forces have been collected to oppose the fiery attack. Satan is very anxious to make an end of the Earth, in order to concentrate his forces

on the Subtle World, which cannot be destroyed in the same way as Earth. Thus the Proprietor of Earth, through present treachery, is betraying the Earth. He is a poor Proprietor in that he cultivated such a nature within himself. He causes Us double labor by keeping up the fires of chaos. Urusvati has seen not a few apparatus; but over and above them stands psychic energy, and therefore We are so careful with it just now.

220. Fiery labor is indeed full of dangers. Urusvati already knows how fiery tension acts. Not only in the earthly body but also in the subtle, it is impossible to withstand for long such tension. Besides, We focus the vortex upon Ourselves, so that a discharged arrow will strike in a center of tension. This method of focusing is employed by Us everywhere. On it is also based the "Tactica Adversa"; from it flow the drops of perspiration, about which you know. But in all, centering is preferable to scattering.

The apparatus which were seen by Urusvati are of enormous force; they are condensers of fiery tension. Thence comes the idea of the swastika. Scholars must review the ancient signs; in them will be found hints of many of Our apparatus.

In the case of such a special problem as that of Earth, chaos represents a great danger.

222. Urusvati has again taken part in fiery labor. To a perceptible extent the inner fire has also appeared externally. It is evident that each approach to the intensified energy burdens the physical organs. Only self-sacrificing spirits can render help. It must be understood that the extraordinary tension indicates agitation of the elements. One must rally all forces in order to preserve

concordance with the Fiery Forces. Verily, there are many black stars. Each day only serves to complicate events.

Fiery World III

128. Many things which it is customary to consider as phenomena may be explained simply as transmutation of one of the centers. How strongly then does create the spirit of the Agni Yogi whose centers have been kindled by sacred fire! Thus, on the path to the Fiery World it is possible to penetrate into the powerful activity of the Agni Yogi. Let us reverence the Mother of Agni Yoga. I have spoken.

134. Therefore, so flamingly beautiful is the task of clarifying the Teaching. It never has happened that the Teaching was affirmed without a fiery clarifier. This task also may be called a sacrificial one. Only a spirit closest in heart can take upon himself this mission. Only a unified consciousness can know the affirmation of Truth. Only a unified consciousness can perceive how to give clarification to the Teaching. We are all, in turn, affirmed as Lawgivers and Clarifiers—this is the Highest Law. The ocean of the Teaching is given only to the nearest one. Humanity suffers so greatly from egoism and self-conceit that it is indispensable to affirm the closest source. Thus, let the heart feel and know in its depths that through the Mother of Agni Yoga is given to the World My Fiery Message. It is essential that the depths of the heart perceive this fiery Truth on all paths.

163. The lightning which cleaves space creates purification of the spheres. Each cosmic manifestation transmutes those energies which must be reworked. In the Cosmic Laboratory are many means of spatial discharges.

Purification is a necessary process in the Cosmos. Knowing the unity of Macrocosm and microcosm, one must find understanding of each process. Who will transmute the spirit of humanity? We say—the lightning of the Spirit of the Bearer of Fire. Who will let fly the cosmic arrow for the destruction of evil? Who will take up the task of cleansing the entrusted Banners? Rightly has been called to mind the Sword of Christ. When cosmic energies are tensed in fiery might, and purifying lightnings are making space tremble, the Fiery Spirit creates correspondingly. The World suffers from halfway measures and suffocates from indulgences—yes, yes, yes! Lightning of the spirit can cleanse space. Lightning of the spirit can make manifest the far-off worlds. Lightning of the spirit can bestow a wonderful future, for lightning of the spirit saturates space with fiery energies. Who will manifest the prophetic fire of purification? Only the Co-worker of Cosmic Forces, only the Co-worker of the Forces of Light. To Her, Co-worker of the Cosmic Forces, Fellow-traveler of the Forces of Light, have I ordained the lightning of the spirit. To Her has been given the right to create with the Cosmic Sword. To Her has been given the Fiery Heart—let the Light be of the lightning of Beauty—yes, yes, yes! I have spoken.

173. There exist many different means for the rarefaction of the dense body. Indeed, each fine thought must be regarded as a fiery manifestation; therefore it is necessary to accustom oneself to think fierily. Rarefaction of the dense physical body must also lie understood from the spiritual point of view, because, while dwelling in a dense body, it is still possible not to manifest coarseness. The Agni Yogi, who has passed through fiery

43

baptism and fiery transmutation, no longer dwells in a dense body, because when the body admits the fiery currents, its whole substance is changed. The basis of this experience of fiery transmutation of the centers is this rarefaction. True, only to the subtle is the subtle accessible, and science of the future will study the subtle body. The ever-increasing fiery manifestations, while directing the spirit into the Higher Worlds, make the earthly spheres burdensome. Let us remember that the subtle is accessible only to the subtle, and let us reverence the Mother of Agni Yoga.

179. Fluids of the fiery heart and spirit nourish the protective net. The fiery centers are a most powerful panacea. The Agni Yogi, being affirmed in the might of fiery energy, possesses the power of the Light; therefore, let us not be surprised if the heart saturated with higher Fire knows nothing of whisperings and temptations. The fluids of such a heart act as purifying energies in space. Currents of the subtle fluids saturate at enormous distances, serving as powerful discharging agents. For example, when the solar plexus is tense, the heart is sending to a far distant point its purifying energies. For example, if absentation is noticed, it means that divisibility of the spirit is in creative process. Pulsations in the extremities and in the heart denote sendings of fiery projectiles. Let us subtly refer to the different manifestations of the spatial creativeness of the powerful Agni Yogi. These cosmic sendings are affirmed by Our Tara, who has taken upon herself the whole achievement of Beauty and Fire.

185. Everything great enters imperceptibly and powerfully into life. The manifestation of Cosmic Right like-

wise enters fierily into life. Invisibly is space saturated; thus powerfully are the fiery threads stretched forth. But when the hour of entrance comes, fiery might will flash out with all the manifested rays of Beauty. Therefore I affirm how vitally necessary it is to understand the power of that great fiery force which is incarnated in the Mother of Agni Yoga. In awesome immensity the threshold draws near; thus a great Mystery enters life.

187. Resounding on the cosmic note can be transmitted spatially to the spirit which perceives the subtle currents. Among the subtle manifestations of such reverberations of the spirit, those which are audible to the fiery spirit must be especially noticed. How vital it is to harken to that apparently inaudible tone which can transmit to the spirit spatial joy or anguish. The manifestation of inexplicable anguish can derive from the sounding of a spatial tone. The subtle organism of this bearer of Fires shudders from these notes of space. The physical ear cannot hear it, but the subtle hearing detects that which is inaudible to the ear and receives it in the heart. Therefore, the striving spirit is a creator in unison with the Cosmos, and knows the cosmic soundings which intensify space. In them is contained summons or call; in them is victory or battle; in them is sorrow or joy. Verily, he who knows these soundings, and experiences the joy and anguish of communion with space, may be called a great Fire- bearer. To this the fiery heart of the Mother of Agni Yoga bears witness. Thus let us remember the great unified Heart.

211. Precisely as Urusvati has said—the fulfillment of one's own duty. Precisely the distribution of assignments in the Cosmos upholds the foundations, and the

Hierarchic Chain maintains equilibrium. There is in the Cosmos one great action which admits of a unified karma, but inasmuch as this is held secret in the Cosmos, the confluence of karma is a solution of Higher Forces. The fiery consciousness and heart can coalesce and bear that Burden of the World, and this will be consecration for the new construction which has been ordained in the Cosmos. The manifestation of the Cosmic Magnet must be saturated with the creativeness of spirit and heart. Thus is affirmed a joint karma. This must be understood as a Higher Token. But when the law of higher significance is applied to daily conditions, this is contrary to Cosmic Ordination. Therefore, on the path to the Fiery World let us be imbued with the significance of the higher uniting of karma.

216. Realization of responsibility for the spirit and for religion has been put by humanity in the last place. The tribunal of regulated society is concerned with preserving the physical body, making mangling of the body liable to prosecution. But existing laws and temples do not concern themselves with the millions who have been mangled in spirit. With justice has Urusvati pointed out the stem responsibility which religions must bear. The uniting function of religion truly has not been awakened on the planet. That sacred power of the Earth, instead of uplifting, has been turned by mankind into production of that obvious disunity which is as a cleaving sword. And priests, and Brahmins, and temple servitors all have distorted the cosmic ordainment. Verily, only affirmation of the true designation will impel the spirit to the higher understanding of the great Cosmic Right. Thus let us strive for the great responsibility for the spirit and for

religion. So much must be purified in the Teachings of the World! The labor of strivingly purifying religions will result in a new consciousness. On the path to the Fiery World let us affirm the Bearers of Fiery Purification.

261. When constructing, one must remember about great correlation. Those who have adhered to the Source of Light must understand that burning of the spirit is beauty and shield in the service of Good. But only those bringing beauty know all the greatness of Service. Therefore it is necessary to note those who defame the manifestation of the Teaching. Many more slanderers of the Teaching can be found among those who have adhered to the Path than among the open enemies. You have pointed out with reason the misunderstandings that inflict blows upon the Shield. Actually it is an application of unfit manifestations. Who will be a follower, if the Teaching is merely an abstraction? It is possible to trace each deplorable consequence precisely as a neglect of understanding of the Living Ethics. Fiery is the heart which knows the affirmation of Service with the Teaching. I manifest as My Will the installation of the Living Ethics and the purification of the Teaching. Without this there is no path to the Fiery World. The greatest task is to affirm a new subtle consciousness. My Will transmits to the Tara My Covenants.

277. When hostile forces disclose an assault, it is needful to think about foresight. The servitors of Light must realize that actually not only do the hostile forces breed treachery, but the menace of treachery and destruction lies precisely in omissions and in slumber. Rightly has she who guides under the Star of the Mother of the World spoken about the fact that a leader values truth, for on

the field of battle it is important to know which swords have been sharpened. Only selfhood impels the spirit to the suppressing of truth.

288. Each of Urusvati's centers is so sensitive to catastrophes. Hence the heart absorbs all energies as in a spatial funnel, feeling each vibration. Therefore the sunlike heart helps in the purification of space. The impetuous heart goes to meet each fiery energy half-way. Such impetuousness is possible only through fiery self-activity, which is attained on a highest step of fiery transmutation. Therefore each cosmic vibration is felt so sharply. When We indicate earthquakes, one should not always expect external manifestations. One must first of all bear in mind those tremors which take place in the depths. Therefore, those pangs which are felt so deeply by the centers have a relationship to the depths of the Earth. Thus, the sunlike heart senses all fiery manifestations.

308. Fiery energies, being drawn into tension by some center, can often cause enhanced actions of the energies of this center. Partial action of energies gives a center the power to manifest partially. These tensions lead to those partial manifestations which bring into error consciousnesses of small discrimination. With reason has Urusvati pointed out those manifestations, evoked by the tension of one center, which lead to psychism. Truly, each opening, saturation or irritation of the centers gives a sharp direction to the fiery energy; but only conformity between the state of the organism and the spiritual awakening produces, as an inevitable effect, the opening of the centers in highest tension. A partial pressure will produce a partial attainment, which may

prove to be a very dangerous manifestation. On the path to the Fiery World let us strive to realize the higher tension of fiery energy.

398. The fire which menaced the Mother of Agni Yoga on the heights was a synthetic discharge of spatial fire. Besides fiery transmutation, this fire, as it were, transmuted all the surrounding atmosphere. This occult and physical fire, verily, expiated all the manifestations which had been accumulated in that space. The subtle organism has many functions. The functions of the fiery spirit are so diverse. The Agni Yogi unburdens space and absorbs all emanations. He is a mighty warrior, battling with darkness, and he is that power which the dark pack is endeavoring to destroy.

Aum

544. It is not at all easy to be the Mother of Agni Yoga. Only in the course of time will people appreciate all the selflessness which is indispensable for proclaiming the fiery might.

Selections from the

LETTERS OF HELENA ROERICH

on

- AGNI YOGA, THE TEACHING OF LIVING ETHICS
- AGNI YOGIS
- AMRITA
- BROTHERS OF HUMANITY
- CHALICE
- EPOCH OF MAITREYA
- FOHAT
- GURU
- MATERIA LUCIDA
- MATERIA MATRIX
- TARA

AGNI YOGA

13 October 1929. Each one must find the key to the Teaching in his own heart. The understanding of the Teaching of Life should inaugurate the creativeness of the spirit. The Image of the Teacher can give an enlightened path toward cosmic space. Thus, when we accept within our hearts the chosen Image, do not our hearts become aflame with love toward all beings? The creative Materia Lucida serves as embodiment for the high spirit, but this energy is attracted through love. The whole Cosmos is upheld by love. Love is the greatest magnet. (*Letters Of Helena Roerich*. Vol. I, New York, Agni Yoga Society, 2017, p. 20).

3 December 1930. Now as regards Agni Yoga. How can we interpret Agni Yoga if we do not broaden our consciousness? All the words about it and about its achievements will be void of conviction if we ourselves do not light the fires of our own hearts. Someone writes about the necessity of tolerance toward every interpretation. This idea is correct. It is, however, necessary to learn how to make each individual interpretation correctly understood. (*Ibid.*, p.52)

7 June 1934. You may call the Teaching "The Living Ethics," if you would rather avoid the Eastern terminology, which sounds strange to some people. (*Ibid.*, p.212)

30 June 1934. And now I shall deal with the question about reading other books in general. Apparently this question worries everybody. Of course there are no objections against reading books concerning various branches of knowledge, art and spirituality, for one should always extend one's knowledge. But it is quite essential to learn to discriminate as regards quality. Thus, I always warn against pseudo-occult books. And when one has the possibility of obtaining all the treasures from the books of the Teaching of Life, which deal with all the problems of life and show new ways of knowledge, and when one has the chance of becoming acquainted with *The Mahatma Letters* ... as well as with not a few works by H. P. Blavatsky, then the reading of lesser books will be a waste of time. With few exceptions, these other books are often a mere echo— frequently erroneous—of the above-mentioned ones. For instance, *Esoteric Buddhism*, by A. P. Sinnett, is based entirely on the letters from the Mahatmas received by Sinnett through H. P. Blavatsky. But all these letters are much more complete in the book, *Mahatma Letters*. I personally always advise the reading of Eastern philosophy, provided, of course, that it is not distorted in translation.

It would be excellent if all the co-workers could become acquainted with the *Foundations of Buddhism*, the Upanishads, the Bhagavad-Gita, the Teachings of Confucius, Lao Tze, Zoroaster, Hermes, and others.... If correctly understood, these Teachings can strengthen the consciousness and help in the assimilation of the Teaching of Living Ethics. I always recommend the reading of the books of Vivekananda and the Gospel of Ramakrishna. I also love the four volumes dedicated to the lives of Ramakrishna and Vivekananda. When reading these books, one is fascinated by the refinement of feeling and thoughts of the East. Fine are the works of Sister Nivedita about India and Vivekananda, who was her teacher. Altogether, there are many beautiful Eastern books. . . .

If the readers of the Teaching of Life, or the Living Ethics, would think more profoundly about all the problems of life, about all new domains of knowledge which are discussed therein, if they would but decide to study them thoroughly, there would be enough material not only for one life, but for several. But usually people read with their eyes, not with their hearts, and that is why the most remarkable indications, the greatest revelations, just slide over their consciousness without leaving the slightest trace. I, having the key to so many of the statements in the books of the Teaching, sadly realize this. These books give direction to the whole mentality; they point out the new domains; they set the new signposts for all scientific research. These books are so vital, so essential, because they lead to the future. The books of the Teaching should be a perpetual source of knowledge to the scientist whose consciousness is not obscured by prejudices. (*Ibid.*, p.222-224)

17 August 1934. As I have mentioned already many times, it is most important to bring into life the educational and cultural ideas without insisting upon, or forcing on people, the books of the Teaching. The more so as the principles and ideas expressed in the Teaching do not bear any specific stamp, and all of them can very well enter into a general concept of Living Ethics. Many themes for lectures and essays could be borrowed from the Teaching of Life. Thus, the fundamental rule must be not to proclaim and not to force. While it is important to raise the consciousness of those who are able to go forward in step with evolution, it should he done by simple methods and images, gradually broadening the concepts until they reach full scope. Of course, I well understand that it is difficult constantly to step down to the level of the majority, but the great joy of the possibility of perpetually receiving from the limitless source of knowledge and beauty is left to us. (*Ibid.*, p.251)

1 February 1935. I strongly recommend that you read the works of the great Origen, that brilliant expounder of the true Teaching of Christ. Incidentally, the Western Church has now commenced to study his works, as the more informed clergy now understands that the church with its dead dogma has come to an impasse and can no longer maintain its influence with the new consciousness of the broad masses, who, first of all, demand logic and flexibility of laws. (*Ibid.*, p.354)

AGNI YOGIS

11 September 1929. People will come to you with questions and indications about various psychic and mediumistic phenomena, considering them as manifestations of Agni Yoga. Therefore, I shall try to clarify this difference...

If it may be so expressed, it is usually the lowest centers of the medium that act by their primitive tension. Often it is a forced phenomenon, which does not lead to the opening of the centers but merely toward their temporary irritation. But the fires of the Agni Yogi are due to the kindling of the highest centers, which really are opened.

Strictly speaking, there are no lower centers, and the Agni Yogi has his "lower" centers transmuted by the finest fires. But this transmutation takes place after the kindling of the highest centers, and then all the "lower" centers are subordinated to the solar plexus. We must also remember that the gradation of these fires, or rather their quality, is infinitely perfected, just as everything else in the Cosmos. But one principle is beyond doubt in determining the Agni Yogi—it is the principle of synthesis. To kindle the fires without the Synthesis of the Chalice is impossible. By this principle you can already determine the quality of the fires.

So you have the main indication by which you can distinguish the manifestations of the ignition of the centers from the lower psychic manifestations. "An Agni Yogi is the carrier of the Synthesis of the Chalice—by this indication you can judge." Therefore, fill your Chalices with the realization of beauty, with the true knowledge of the wisdom of the Teaching of Life, and with the assimilation of it in your heart, and remember that the heart is a great magnet which attracts all knowledge, all possibilities, and all achievements. You should remember also that there is nothing forced in the manifestations of an Agni Yogi, as the Agni Yogi is his own laboratory. He, himself, by the force of his spirit, transforms his fires. The Teacher gives the Indications of the Teaching for broadening the consciousness, but the pupil himself must apply it. The Teacher watches over the process of igniting by covering the centers with layers of soma when the ignition threatens to become a conflagration. But without the participation of the spirit of the pupil no transmutation is possible. (*Ibid.*, p.26-28)

1 August 1934. Note that soma is not the ethereal body. Soma is a subtle secretion of the glands which can create a sort of protective net for the centers. Therefore, with such protection the transmutation of the centers may be continued, as the insulation of the centers makes this transmutation less dangerous. Even under the snow some plants live and grow. Sometimes the most wonderful plants develop under the pure snow. Thus, soma offers protection against fire. (*Ibid.*, p.238)

AMRITA

1929. You, my young friends, who have approached art and creation, you should be able to utilize your gifts as a condensation of your forces; for sound and color, thought and rhythm are the foundations of the Universe and of our existence. Sound and color, knowledge and creation are the chalice of Amrita, the chalice of Immortality! (*Ibid.*, p.12)

17 August 1930. So many disappointments, so many failures would have been avoided had the Teaching and all the indications been applied in a literal sense in everyday life. By giving us understanding of life, understanding of the foundations of existence, the Teaching brings us, if there is application in full consciousness of all that is given, to fiery purification or transmutation of our centers into the higher fires, and thus gives us the chalice of Amrita. (*Ibid.*, p.41)

11 January 1933. Reaching a state of conscious continuity of existence, or of the preservation of a complete consciousness in all the bodies and in all the spheres, is the greatest achievement of the Arhat. This is what is called Amrita, or true immortality. That is why all the efforts of the Great Teachers are directed toward the broadening of the consciousness of humanity, the development of the mental body, and the awakening of the higher aspiration for the creating of the magnetic current which uplifts the spirit into the higher spheres. (*Ibid.*, p.344)

BROTHERS OF HUMANITY

20 December 1934. You may tell your interrogators that the true Teaching never repudiates the foundations of the most ancient Covenants, and that these foundations are based on reverence to the Great Hierarchy. Without the bond with the Hierarchy of Light, our destiny is as that of a kitten at sea. What can exist without the Leading Concept? Verily, the Concept of Hierarchy is a Cosmic Concept and a Cosmic Law. The whole Universe is nourished and sustained under this Fiery Law. Therefore, every teaching that denies this Principle is a false teaching.

Regarding initiations, I may say that in life there are many degrees of initiation, and each one who knows a little more than his neighbor is already initiated into something. Also, please distinguish thoroughly between the White Brothers, Members of the Himalayan Community, and the ordinary white brothers, who are people following the Teaching of Light.

The majority of the Great Brothers are now using densified subtle bodies. And Those who are still in their physical bodies are gathered now in the main Stronghold. All the Ashrams in Tibet are hidden in closed, impassable defiles. The dreadful effluvia of the earthly atmosphere does not encourage the presence of the Great Teachers among people. Moreover, at the moment their work does not require their physical presence. Such terms as "Initiate," "Adept," "White Brother" are terribly profaned! It would be a good thing to ponder upon the words of the Great Teacher K. H.: "An Adept is the rarest flower of a whole series of generations of seekers." Yet, indeed, how many times this flower has been born among the host of these self-sacrificing Sages! Thus, let us manifest here the highest care, and let us not profane the greatest concepts! It is truly impossible to imagine the entire majesty of an Arhat of the Hierarchy of Light! It cannot be comprehended by our limited minds and imagination. Only the tremor of the heart will indicate the spiritual exaltation of a devoted disciple, who feels the approaching Ray of the Teacher of Light! (*Ibid.*, 337)

12 April 1935. Among the Great Teachers, the manifestation of the Eye of Dangma is especially valued. This is not clairvoyance, as generally understood, but the straight-knowledge accumulated in the Chalice during thousands of lives and self-sacrificing experiences. The goal of this accumulation is to achieve a great destiny and become a full Arhat, or Man-God. (*Ibid.*, p.393)

20 April 1935. Not a single Great Teacher of Humanity has left our solar system. Moreover, They have not even left the spheres which surround our planet. On the contrary, They are now nearer to us than ever, as the fury of Armageddon requires the tension of all the Forces of the Hierarchy of Light. But even if there were no Armageddon, all these Highest Spirits would continue their perfecting on other higher spheres and planets still within the boundaries of our solar system. Earth is not the highest planet in our solar system. The High Spirits came to our planet from a higher planet for the acceleration of the evolution of our humanity. But since their planet has not as yet completed the entire cycle of its evolution, They will return there when the cycle will be in conformity with their spiritual state. (*Ibid.*, p.401)

31 May 1935. Buddha held woman in the greatest esteem, and stated that she could achieve, as well as man, the highest degrees of Arhatship. Verily, the same fire of spirit, the same monad is aflame in woman as in man; the psychic apparatus of woman is more subtle than that of man. That is why in ancient Egypt the high priestesses of Isis transmitted the orders of the Goddess to the Hierophants, but never vice versa....

True history, and especially true knowledge, will reveal many astonishing pages and real facts. Let us recollect these great words: "It could be said that not a single Covenant has reached us without distortion. Endless are the alterations and distortions which have appeared in the translations of the great writers." How terribly distorted are the works of the first Fathers of Christianity. Let us take, for instance, the great Origen. Do we not have an example of such distortion in the preface to his works written by his disciple? Verily, the deeper we ponder upon the origins of all the Teachings, the more clearly is their oneness and grandeur manifested. Therefore, in our ignorance, let us not accuse the great Founders of the Teachings who assuredly knew about the great law of Equilibrium of the Elements. In antiquity the last and highest Initiation was connected with this illumination and knowledge. The entire mystery, the whole beauty of Be-ness was revealed to the soul illumined by the highest Light. Even in distorted Hinduism there are preserved some hints of the significance of the Feminine Element. And even up to the present day, the most sacred ritual cannot be performed by a Brahmin without the participation of his wife.

Christ also asserted the equality of the Elements; but dark were the followers of his disciples, and this darkness increased, so to speak, not in arithmetic but in geometric progression.

Likewise, Zoroaster highly esteemed the Feminine Element, and in his Covenants one may find remarkable hints as to the grandeur of Cosmic Love. (*Ibid.*, 420-421)

CHALICE

3 December 1930. The accumulation of the precipitation of energies does not take place in just a single life. Thousands of years are necessary for filling the Chalice. So essential are the continuous, never-interrupted, benevolent strivings, which deposit the priceless treasures in our treasury. People possessing great accumulations of the Chalice are the treasures of nations. Sometimes very little is needed in order to complete the filling of the Chalice, and this little could be completed in one self-denying life. But by carelessness people postpone the achievement, and by this they throw themselves back. Nobody and nothing can stop eternal movement and the transmutation of energies. There exist only two possibilities: either to strive ahead or to fall back. But who would want to vow himself to retrogression —in other words, to unite himself with cosmic waste? Striving is the great moving power for all beings! (*Ibid.*, 51-52)

7 June 1934. The tension mentioned in the Teaching is not a physical overstraining but *a vigilance and mobility of consciousness.* This in turn influences our vitality, as the awakened, broadened consciousness makes a person twice as strong. (However, vigilance of consciousness does not mean that one should try to do without sleep.) The centers also can be opened only in the cases where the consciousness is broadened. But the opening of the centers is not the final achievement; afterwards comes their fiery transmutation. The path of discipleship is not as simple as many think. It is made easier for those who have striven to fill their Chalice. Therefore, do not expect opened centers in every kind of psychic manifestation. Even should there be a slight opening of one of the centers, there are such endless gradations of these partially opened centers! Therefore, remember what is said in the Teaching about "the rings of keen sight and hearing." (*Ibid.*, p.212)

8 May 1933. Straight-knowledge is knowledge and experience accumulated in our Chalice. It is the so-called intuition, but of an extremely high quality. (*Ibid.*, p.412)

EPOCH OF MAITREYA

8 August 1934. The Great Spirit who is at the head of the New Cycle must contain within Himself all synthesis, all the greatest Images of the past Cycle. That is why the Synthesis of Maitreya includes all the Rays. (*Ibid.*, p.245)

8 March 1935. The equilibrium of the elements is a foundation of Life, and the violation of this law leads to destruction. And now the Great Teachers will affirm the rights of woman. Therefore, the coming epoch will be not only an epoch of great cooperation, it will also be the epoch of Woman. Woman will have to be armed with courage, and, first of all, she will have to restrain her heart from unwise giving, for there must be the Golden Balance in everything. Woman must affirm herself, and that is why the Sword of Spirit is given precisely into the hands of woman. In the East this epoch is noted as the epoch of Maitreya, the epoch of Great Compassion, and the epoch of the Mother of the World. (*Ibid.*, p.376)

8 May 1935. Truly, the women must sacredly guard the chalice entrusted to them: the moving of the consciousness and the saving of the world. The Epoch of Maitreya is the epoch of Woman.

Let our every day be dedicated to the service of the Great Movement. (*Ibid.*, p.416)

FOHAT

20 April 1935. Fohat is the subtlest fiery energy, and if it contacts an unprepared organism it may burn and cause torturous fiery death. I myself saw Fohat with my physical eyes, and was full of wonder at the splitting of the sun rays into millions of luminous sparks of Fohat. Afterwards I suffered a slight singeing of the centers. Likewise, I saw the crystal of Materia Lucida. All this was shown to me by the Great Teacher. I also was twice on the verge of fiery death, and was saved by the Rays of the Great Teacher. But this degree of experience is rather rare and one has to go through the preparatory degrees of fiery manifestation, otherwise an inopportune death would result. When the right moment comes for the assimilation of the higher fiery energies, the events of life are so arranged that the disciple comes to the right place where such experience can be given. If a disciple is ready, nothing can prevent him from receiving what is well deserved. As it is said in the Teaching, "each one will allot to himself his share." (*Ibid.*, p.402)

GURU

11 August 1934. You ask, "Is it necessary to have an earthly teacher until one is accepted as a close disciple by the Great Master?" But let me remind you that you yourself arrange special groups and appoint the instructors! Why do you act in this way? Are you not doing this for a better assimilation of the first steps of the Teaching, and consequently for further progress? And what would you call such instructors? Are they not also earthly teachers? And were not the great Founders of religions and the great philosophers, in their time, just "earthly teachers"? And did not people scoff and revolt against them? And now they are all elevated to the status of Gods and Great Illuminati by the very same adversaries!

Have you ever thought why among the Great Community, or Brotherhood, we meet mostly those who are Easterners by birth? Has it not something to do with the very character of the people of the East, a character which possesses special qualities? Exactly so. And the first of these qualities, which has been impressed upon the consciousness of the people for centuries, is precisely the quality of devotion to the Guru! In the East, the bond between the disciple and the Guru is considered even now to be the most sacred, and above all blood relationships. And occultly, it is quite correct because the Guru creates the consciousness of the real man, the inner man who is the carrier of his karma; and by so doing the Guru takes responsibility even for a part of the karma of his disciple. Therefore, the selecting of disciples as well as of a Teacher must be done with great thoughtfulness and care.

But those who are far from the understanding of

the sacred conception of discipleship must not be forced by us. Let them go their own way. The shortest way—the way of the heart—is rarely reached, or rather rarely chosen. It requires a great degree of devotion, this rarest quality of nobility, which in our age has all sorts of substitutes, and which is being chiefly replaced by devotion to the "golden calf." (*Ibid.*, p.247-248)

MATERIA LUCIDA

8 May 1935. Materia Lucida is the degree of the Primary Matter on the astral plane, and it is still attainable for investigation, but of course having its own degrees or gradations. (*Ibid.*, p.413)

MATERIA MATRIX

8 May 1935. Materia Matrix is beyond the astral plane, and is an equivalent of Mulaprakriti, Akasha, Primary Substance—the subtlest, super-sensuous, ethereal substance, which fills the whole of space— the Mysterium Magnum of the alchemists. (*Ibid.*, p.413)

TARA

16 January 1935. Tara is a goddess, the feminine equivalent of the Arhat, or a Sister of the White Brotherhood. But please do not be too much interested in the names of various initiations; this will not lead you anywhere. In ancient times, each religio-philosophical school or sacred brotherhood had its own gradations or degrees, and had special names for them. But you may be sure that the true degrees were not designated by the names we now see in books. If you are interested in this, take the beautiful definitions of the degrees of spiritual advancement given in *Agni Yoga*. Indeed, among some who study occultism, there are those who are convinced that the Sun-initiation takes place on the physical sun! All degrees of initiation are in ourselves. When a disciple is ready, he receives a Ray of Illumination, which corresponds with the degree of purification he has achieved, as well as of the broadening of his consciousness and the fiery transmutation of his centers. (*Ibid.*, p.352)

AGNI YOGA SERIES

Leaves of Morya's Garden I (The Call) 1924

Leaves of Morya's Garden II (Illumination) 1925

New Era Community 1926

Signs of Agni Yoga

Agni Yoga 1929

Infinity I 1930

Infinity II 1930

Hierarchy 1931

Heart 1932

Fiery World I 1933

Fiery World II 1934

Fiery World III 1935

Aum 1936

Brotherhood 1937

Supermundane (in 3 volumes) 1938

Letters of Helena Roerich, Vol. I 1929-1935

Letters of Helena Roerich, Vol. II 1935-1939

AGNI YOGA SOCIETY
www.agniyoga.org

www.ingramcontent.com/pod-product-compliance
Lightning Source LLC
Chambersburg PA
CBHW072156020426
42334CB00018B/2032